MW01712129

SPHEROCYTOSIS SIMPLY EXPLAINED

SPHEROCYTOSIS SIMPLY EXPLAINED

Chris Greenaway

Published by Zinc Tree Press
Cambridge

This book is not intended to be medical advice. You should seek the advice of a medical practioner before starting, stopping or altering any treatment. Your doctor can provide personal care based on your medical history, this book cannot. The publisher and author disclaim liability for any medical outcomes that may occur as a result of information contained in this book. This book does not contain all available information on the subject.

This edition published in Great Britain in 2012 by
Zinc Tree Press
Cambridge

1 3 5 7 9 10 8 6 4 2

ISBN-13 978-0-9571945-0-2
ISBN-10 0-9571945-0-1

Contents

Introduction

Overview

Spherocytosis is a medical condition. If you have it, then your red blood cells are an unusual shape.

The general population have red blood cells that are biconcave, their red blood cells look a bit like a ring doughnut with the hole in the middle filled in. Those with spherocytosis have red blood cells that resemble a ball or sphere.

The spherical shape occurs because a protein that forms part of the structure of a red blood cell is different to normal. A genetic mutation is the usual reason for this, but it can also happen with some autoimmune diseases where the body degrades its own red blood cells.

When spherocytosis is caused by a genetic mutation, it is known as hereditary spherocytosis. This occurs at an incidence of around 1 in 2,000. This level of incidence is typical across a variety of ethnic backgrounds.

The spherical red blood cells are called spherocytes. Normal, biconcave red blood cells typically survive for around 120 days, whereas spherocytes only last for about 20 days.

The destruction of red blood cells is called hemolysis. When the spherocytes pass through a narrow point in the spleen they are trapped and put under stress. While they are trapped they come under attack from immune cells. The extra stress on the red blood cells causes damage, which can attract the immune cells.

The higher rate of hemolysis (red blood cell break down) in those with spherocytosis leads to two changes that potentially cause symptoms: fewer red blood cells and higher levels of red blood cell break down products. The severity of symptoms is directly related to the severity of these changes.

Having fewer red blood cells is called anemia. It lowers the body's ability to transport oxygen round the body. This can lead to a paler skin colour and fatigue.

In extreme cases, the body does not get an adequate level of oxygen. This is known as hypoxia and it can cause headaches, shortness of breath, lowered consciousness or death.

Bilirubin is the hemolysis product that causes the most significant problems.

A high level of bilirubin in the blood turns the skin and the whites of the eyes turn yellow. This is known as jaundice. The whites of the eyes are usually the first place this yellowing can be seen. Jaundice caused by hemolysis does not generally cause any problems other than the yellowing, except in infants, where it can cause brain damage.

If levels of bilirubin are higher than normal over an extended period of time, as is often the case with spherocytosis, this can lead to a build up of bilirubin in the gallbladder and consequently an increased risk of gallstones.

A gallstone that enters any of the ducts leading away from the gallbladder is extremely painful and, if a duct becomes blocked, life threatening conditions can quickly develop.

Some infections can temporarily increase the severity of symptoms in someone with spherocytosis. Red blood cell production can stop, or hemolysis can be much higher. Both can lead to dangerous levels of anemia.

Because those with spherocytosis have a higher level of hemolysis, the spleen can become enlarged due to the increased demands on it. Often the spleen becomes large enough for a doctor to feel it during a physical examination of the abdomen.

There are a wide range of tests to confirm a diagnosis of hereditary spherocytosis including the peripheral blood smear, cryohemolysis test and EMA binding test. Tests vary in their accuracy, availability, cost and ease of administration. A child should be tested at birth if either parent is known to have spherocytosis.

The recommended treatment for spherocytosis depends on the severity of symptoms.

For those with a relatively mild condition, an increase in the intake of folate may be helpful. Folate is used by the body to create new red blood cells. Folic acid is a form of folate that can be taken as a tablet.

If you take folic acid supplements then you should also consider taking vitamin B12. A lack of B12 can cause anemia and neurological damage. Taking folic acid masks anemia that results from a B12 deficiency, so it is likely that the deficiency would only be detected at a much later stage, once irreversible neurological damage had already occurred.

Where the symptoms of spherocytosis are more severe, the spleen can be removed (splenectomy). Typically, this significantly reduces or eliminates most problems related to spherocytosis. However, there are relatively rare, but serious, complications associated with having no spleen, including sepsis (blood poisoning) which can be fatal. Because of this, pneumococcal vaccines and influenza vaccines should be given regularly to those with no spleen.

If a person with spherocytosis is suffering from a pronounced anemia due to a low number of red blood cells then blood transfusions may be necessary. However, numerous blood transfusions can raise levels of iron because the body does not easily dispose of the extra metal ions that are introduced with the transfused blood. This can lead to hemochromatosis, a serious condition that can cause liver damage. Those with spherocytosis are also at a higher risk, compared to the general population, of having a genetic form of hemochromatosis.

Recent research has indicated that antioxidants may help reduce the hemolysis and so reduce the level of anemia in those with hereditary spherocytosis.

Longer term monitoring of red blood count levels is common

for those with spherocytosis, especially for children or those who still have their spleen.

A test reporting the amount of hemoglobin in the blood indicates the seriousness of the anemia. The result is normally given in grams per decilitre. A normal adult would have between 12 and 17. Someone with mild spherocytosis might have a test result of around 11. Severe cases might have around 6. A result of 4 or 5 would require immediate blood transfusion.

Myths

Myth: If you have spherocytosis you should get a splenectomy.

Truth: There are serious risks associated with having your spleen removed. If you have a relatively mild form of spherocytosis then you are probably better off keeping your spleen.

Myth: Spherocytosis is mostly a disease limited to those of Northern European descent.

Truth: It occurs in around 1 in 2,000 of those of Northern European descent. A similar incidence is found in those of Hispanic, Japanese and African descents.

Myth: Now that you have had your spleen out, you never need to worry about any of this again.

Truth: If you have no spleen, you have a much higher risk from some infections. You should be regularly vaccinated against pneumococcus and influenza.

Myth: Spherocytosis is caused by a dominant gene so your children are likely to inherit it from you.

Truth: Spherocytosis is caused by a variety of gene mutations. Some are dominant, some are recessive. It is far less likely that your children would inherit your spherocytosis if you have a recessive form.

Myth: The recessive form of spherocytosis is more severe.

Truth: There are a variety of mutations that cause recessive spherocytosis. Some give particularly severe symptoms, such as mutations of the α-spectrin gene. Some give relatively mild symptoms, such as mutations of the protein 4.2 gene.

Myth: Splenectomy will completely cure your spherocytosis.

Truth: Those with a severe form of spherocytosis may still have some mild symptoms after splenectomy.

Myth: Your spherocytosis seems mild so you have nothing to worry about.

Truth: Gallstones are a common complication of spherocytosis and potentially very painful. Even those with mild symptoms can get gallstones. They develop slowly, so you may only have symptoms when you get older. If you have spherocytosis, the chance of having gallstones is around 40% at age 20, rising to 80% at age 75.

Myth: If you have spherocytosis, you should be taking iron supplements.

Truth: People with spherocytosis can often suffer from iron overload. Frequently because they are given blood transfusions, but also because they are more likely to have a genetic condition that causes high iron levels. High levels are dangerous and can lead to permanent liver damage.

Myth: If you are taking folic acid every day, you do not need any other supplements.

Truth: Vitamin B12 deficiency can cause both anemia and neurological damage. Taking folic acid can prevent that anemia, but the neurological damage continues and might only be spotted once the damage is irreversible. Consider taking a B12 supplement as well.

Myth: All spherocytosis is hereditary spherocytosis.

Truth: Autoimmune spherocytosis is another form of spherocytosis. The body's immune system damages the red blood cells causing them to become spherical.

Fundamentals

Genetics

Hereditary spherocytosis is a genetic condition.

Genes are a code that the body uses to build proteins. When the sequence of letters in a gene changes this usually causes a different protein to be built. A gene often has variants in the population, known as alleles.

Most people inherit two copies of each gene, one from each parent. Normally, both copies are used to produce protein.

Having the same allele for both copies of a gene is known as homozygous. In this case, that allele determines the individual's phenotype (observable characteristics).

Having two different alleles is called heterozygous. In this case, an allele is said to be dominant if the individual's phenotype is the same as the phenotype that occurs with two copies of that allele.

For example, a mutant gene that causes the resulting protein to block some other process in the body would probably be dominant because this protein will cause a problem regardless of the ability of the normal gene to produce a normal protein.

Alleles that only affect the phenotype when there are two copies (homozygous) are known as recessive.

For example, a mutant gene that causes the resulting protein to be ineffective, but is otherwise harmless, would likely be recessive because the other, normal copy of the gene can produce the normal protein.

Spherocytosis can be caused by a variety of mutant genes, some dominant, others recessive. All of these spherocytosis genes, however, are autosomal which means that there is no specific sex that the genes are associated with. In other words, you can inherit a spherocytosis gene from either your mother or father and you can pass the gene on to any children that you have, boys or girls.

Red blood cells

Red blood cells deliver oxygen to the body. Each one contains a concentrated solution of hemoglobin. Hemoglobin is a molecule that binds to oxygen in the relatively high oxygen concentration of the lungs and then later releases it where oxygen levels are low. About a third of a red blood cell is hemoglobin, most of the rest is water.

Red blood cells are more formally known as erythrocytes. The "erythro" prefix comes from the Greek for red. Red blood cells are red because oxygenated hemoglobin absorbs green and blue light.

There are around 30 trillion red blood cells in the body. Each one has approximately 270 million molecules of hemoglobin. Every molecule of hemoglobin can carry eight atoms of oxygen. That means that the body has a total carrying capacity of about 60 billion trillion oxygen atoms.

A red blood cell lacks the cell components that are normally found inside other cells, such as a nucleus or mitochondria. Consequently, it does not use up the oxygen that it carries, but it is incapable of self-repair.

Red blood cells normally last around 120 days before they are removed by macrophages in the spleen that detect damaged cells. In hereditary spherocytosis, the red blood cells only survive for between 10 and 30 days depending on the severity of the condition.

To replace those that are destroyed, about 2.5 million new red blood cells are created every second. The kidneys detect lowered levels of oxygen and release a biochemical called erythropoietin (also known as EPO) which stimulates stem cells in the red bone marrow to differentiate (become more specialised) into red blood cells, in a process called erythropoiesis.

The new red blood cells are released into the blood stream before they are fully mature. These immature red blood cells are called reticulocytes. Unlike mature red blood cells, reticulocytes still contain some RNA (similar to DNA), that is visible as dark granules under a microscope.

It takes a day or two for a reticulocyte to mature. During this time the red blood cell becomes stronger, it loses surface area and its final shape is formed: biconcave for normal red blood cells; spherical in hereditary spherocytosis.

Normally, about 1% of red blood cells are reticulocytes, but in spherocytosis this figure is substantially higher, around 4% for a mild form of spherocytosis and over 10% in severe cases. This is because red blood cells do not last as long, so younger ones form a larger part of the population.

The rate of red blood cell production increases because the persistent anemia continually prompts the kidneys to produce erythropoietin in an attempt to compensate.

The production of red blood cells stops during an aplastic crisis and this can lead to abnormally low reticulocyte levels.

Structural proteins

Spherocytosis can be caused by mutations in the genes for a variety of structural proteins that are used in the red blood cell membrane.

The cytoskeleton is a relatively rigid structure that supports the cell membrane. It forms a network that approximates a hexagonal lattice. A protein called spectrin forms the arms and a protein called actin forms the junctions (actin is shown as a hexagon in the diagram).

Each arm contains two copies of spectrin pointing in opposite directions and each spectrin molecule is composed of two separate proteins α-spectrin and β-spectrin (respectively shown as

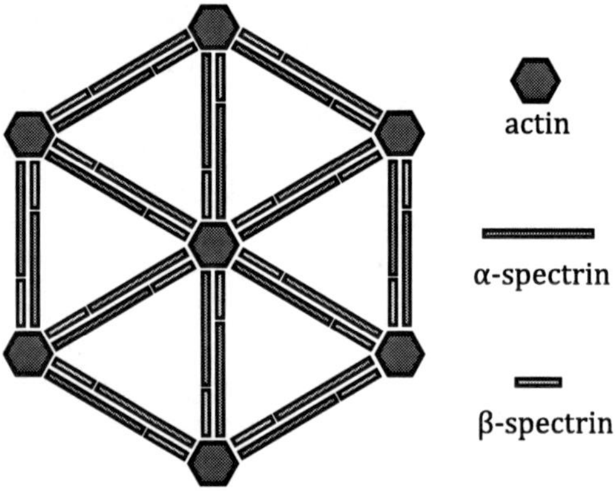

Spectrin-actin network structure

long and short rectangles in the diagram). Spectrin acts like a relatively weak spring and this gives a normal red blood cell the ability to deform and then recover its shape.

A protein called ankyrin attaches the spectrin-actin network to the cell membrane at the spectrin arms. Without the ankyrin holding the spectrin to the cell membrane, the spectrin is not stable.

Band 3 protein (also called anion exchange protein 1 or AE1) makes up around 25% of the surface area of the cell membrane. It is responsible for exchanging chloride and bicarbonate ions across the cell membrane. It also helps stabilise the cell membrane.

Protein 4.2 helps to link the ankyrin and band 3 proteins.

In a red blood cell there are approximately 250,000 spectrin molecules (two for each arm), 125,000 ankyrin molecules (one for each arm), 1.2 million band 3 protein molecules and 200,000 protein 4.2 molecules.

Protein defects in spherocytosis

Mutations in the genes for any one of these structural proteins can cause spherocytosis.

The gene for band 3 protein has around 50 known mutant versions. There are a similar number for the ankyrin gene, around twenty for the β-spectrin gene, a couple for the α-spectrin gene and about eight for the protein 4.2 gene.

This wide range of possible genetic causes of spherocytosis leads to the wide range in severity of the disease.

Mutations of the α-spectrin gene are normally recessive and β-spectrin gene mutations are normally dominant. This is because, in a genetically normal individual, roughly four times more α-spectrin is produced than β-spectrin. Because spectrin is made up of equal quantities of α-spectrin and β-spectrin, a small or moderate drop in α-spectrin production has no impact on the overall amount of spectrin produced. The α-spectrin only becomes a limiting factor when both copies of the gene are affected. Conversely, *any* drop in β-spectrin production has an immediate impact on the overall amount of spectrin produced.

Mutations of the β-spectrin gene are responsible for around 30% of spherocytosis cases and cause mild to moderate symptoms. The α-spectrin gene mutations cause less than 5% of cases, but result in severe symptoms including transfusion dependency. Because the α-spectrin gene is recessive, both copies must be mutated to cause a problem and this is why these cases are more serious, there is no normal copy to produce at least some normal protein.

Mutations of the ankyrin gene are responsible for around 45% of spherocytosis cases. Some mutations of this gene are dominant, some are recessive. Because the ankyrin helps to stabilise the spectrin, any reduction in ankyrin availability has a direct effect on the amount of spectrin that can be incorporated into the cell structure. So mutations of the ankyrin gene typically lead to combined spectrin and ankyrin deficiency in the cell membrane.

Band 3 protein gene mutations are responsible for around 25% of spherocytosis cases and can cause red blood cells to have a mushroom shape. Typically, the mutations of this gene are dominant and cause only mild to moderate symptoms. This protein is also used in the kidney, so mutations of the gene can also cause distal renal tubular acidosis. In this condition, acids are not correctly passed to the urine, potentially causing a range of symptoms including muscle cramps, lethargy, heart arrhythmia and kidney stones.

Protein 4.2 gene mutations are recessive but normally cause only mild symptoms. They make up less than 5% of spherocytosis cases.

Those of Japanese ancestry have a different profile of genetic causes to those of Northern European descent. For the Japanese, protein 4.2 gene mutations make up about 45% of cases, ankyrin gene mutations - 7%, band 3 gene mutations - 25%, and the rest are spectrin gene mutations. In other words, there is a high percentage of the recessive, mild protein 4.2 mutations and a lower percentage of the ankyrin gene mutations.

Incidence and severity

Incidence

Approximately 1 in 2,000 people have some form of hereditary spherocytosis and about 1 in 5,000 have a moderate or severe case. Screening for hereditary spherocytosis has shown that about 1 in 200 people have some form of the condition with no overt symptoms. Around 1 in 70 are silent carriers for a recessive form.

Figures are often given for people of Northern European, or possibly Hispanic, descent as those are the ethnic groups looked at more frequently in studies, but the incidence does not vary strongly across race.

In those of Northern European descent, hereditary spherocytosis is the most common hemolytic anemia. This is true of those of Japanese ancestry as well, although the ratio of the various associated genetic causes is different.

There is also a significant incidence, around 1 in 2,000, in people of African descent, but that ethnic group has other hemolytic anemias that are even more prevalent, such as sickle cell anemia with an incidence of around 1 in 500.

Severity

There is a large range in the severity of hereditary spherocytosis because it is caused by a wide variety of gene mutations. Cases are usually categorised as mild, moderate, moderately severe or severe.

In mild cases, the hemoglobin level is at the low end of normal, or just below, perhaps around 12 g/dl.

Mild forms of spherocytosis may be fully compensated with the body creating new red blood cells fast enough to match the rate at which red blood cells are destroyed. In this situation, there is little or no anemia, but the spherocytosis can still cause other problems, such as gallstones.

In moderate cases of spherocytosis, the hemoglobin level is substantially below normal, between 8 and 12 g/dl. Typically this causes persistent anemia and someone with a moderate form of spherocytosis can get tired or out of breath easily.

In moderately severe cases, the hemoglobin is between 6 and 8 g/dl. This causes serious anemia.

In severe cases, the anemia is life-threatening and regular blood transfusions are required. Hemoglobin is 6 g/dl or below, without transfusion.

The following table shows the frequency with which the different severities of hereditary spherocytosis occur in the population of those with hereditary spherocytosis.

Severity	Frequency
Mild	25%
Moderate	60%
Moderately severe	10%
Severe	5%

Chance of inheriting

Dominant mutations and recessive mutations have different patterns of inheritance. Regardless of whether the mutation is dominant or recessive, the chances of a child inheriting a certain number of mutated alleles depend on the number of mutated alleles each parent has. The five essentially different cases are shown in the table.

	Mutated allele count of parent		Child's chance of mutated allele count		
Case	A	B	2	1	0
A	2	2	100%	0%	0%
B	2	1	50%	50%	0%
C	2	0	0%	100%	0%
D	1	1	25%	50%	25%
E	1	0	0%	50%	50%

Cases C and E in this table correspond to a single parent who has recessive or dominant spherocytosis respectively.

Dominant pattern

Having two copies of a dominant hereditary spherocytosis allele (cases A, B and C in the table) is extremely rare and often incompatible with life. But there have been cases where people have survived this, with transfusion and splenectomy. In this case, every child will inherit dominant hereditary spherocytosis.

Case D, is relatively rare, both parents have dominant hereditary spherocytosis.

Case E, is a typical situation for dominant hereditary spherocytosis, only one parent has it. In this case, any one child has a 50% chance of inheriting dominant hereditary spherocytosis and a 50% chance of being completely clear.

This pattern is often seen as a line of inheritance running through generations.

Recessive pattern

All the different cases shown in the table come into play much more in the recessive pattern.

Those with two mutated alleles have recessive hereditary spherocytosis, those with one are carriers for the condition.

Case A is unusual, both parents have recessive hereditary spherocytosis. All the children will have it too.

Cases A, B and C show how the probabilities shift from 'all children will have recessive hereditary spherocytosis' to 'all children will be carriers', depending on the other partner's status: having recessive hereditary spherocytosis, a carrier or clear.

Case D shows what happens when two carriers have children. Any one child has a 50% chance of being a carrier, a 25% chance of having recessive hereditary spherocytosis and a 25% chance of being completely clear. Typically, parents do not know they are carriers, so when they have a child with spherocytosis it is often a surprise.

Case E shows that any one child of a carrier has a 50% chance of being a carrier, assuming their partner has no hereditary spherocytosis gene.

Determining the pattern

You can be fairly sure about which pattern of hereditary spherocytosis you have by looking at other members of your family. If one of your parents has it, perhaps some siblings, cousins, grandparents and so on, then this is likely to be dominant hereditary spherocytosis.

A genetic test can tell definitively what mutations you and your partner have.

Spleen

Role of the spleen

The spleen is an organ that is sited on the left hand side of the body just under the ribs. It is composed of red pulp and white pulp which gives it purple-mottled-with-grey appearance.

Normally the spleen is around 10cm long but, in those with spherocytosis, the spleen is often enlarged (splenomegaly).

Red pulp contains a fine mesh of blood vessels that filter the blood. White pulp is responsible for aspects of the immune system, including antibody synthesis.

The red pulp filters old or damaged cells and captures antigens to present to the immune system. Antigens are foreign molecules or cells.

Cells that are part of the immune system, called macrophages, swallow red blood cells and antigens and present them to the immune system. There are other cells in the immune system that can capture antigens, such as dendritic cells.

Once a macrophage has swallowed a red blood cell it breaks it down into amino acids, bilirubin and iron. The iron is either stored in the spleen as ferritin or released as into the blood stream as transferrin. The bilirubin is released (attached to albumin) to be processed by the liver.

When an immune system cell captures an antigen, that antigen is presented to lymphocytes in the white pulp. The lymphocytes are responsible for generating antibodies that are adapted to each specific antigen.

The spleen and spherocytosis

The spleen's filtering process requires red blood cells to squeeze through small gaps. The small veins that lead out of the spleen (sinusoids) have pores in them that allow the blood to enter from the red pulp. Red blood cells must deform to fit through the pores.

The spherocytes (spherical red blood cells) do not fit through these pores so easily, so are more likely to be trapped in the red pulp and swallowed by a macrophage or damaged by oxidants from the macrophages.

Normal red blood cells pass through the spleen's filter in approximately 40 seconds, but spherocytes are estimated to take somewhere between 15 minutes to 150 minutes.

The extra mechanical stress that the spherocytes undergo, when trying to fit through the pores, can damage them. This can cause a biochemical that is normally found on the inside of the cell wall, called phosphatidylserine, to become exposed. The macrophages in the spleen recognise the phosphatidylserine and swallow the cell.

Splenectomy

Surgically removing the spleen (splenectomy) usually completely resolves all symptoms associated wth spherocytosis. The red blood cells still retain their spherical shape, but that does not cause any problems once the spleen is no longer present. Someone with a severe case of spherocytosis may still have some mild symptoms remaining after splenectomy.

There are risks associated with having no spleen. Because the spleen is no longer there to mount an immune response, certain bacterial infections can be fatal, for example pneumococcus (which can cause pneumonia).

If someone with no spleen develops signs of an infection, such as a fever, they should seek medical attention immediately. The onset of a life-threatening situation can be very rapid, within hours.

Vaccinations covering a range of serious infections should be administered before the splenectomy is carried out. This should include vaccinations against pneumonia, meningitis and influenza. Adequate precautions against malaria are also needed.

Repeat vaccinations should be given at suitable intervals after splenectomy, for example, once a year for influenza.

Adhering to the vaccination regime requires some dedication, but it is important as these infections can easily kill if you have no spleen.

The spleen is also responsible for removing old platelets (small cells that help blood to clot). After splenectomy, platelet levels rise. This can cause clots to form inside the body leading to numbness, stroke or heart attack. However, it is relatively rare for platelet levels to rise high enough to cause significant problems. The platelet levels typically fall back to normal within a few weeks, but levels can remain high for years. Taking aspirin can help prevent clots from forming.

Given the substantial risks of splenectomy, it should only be carried out where necessary. If possible, it should be delayed in young children as their immune system has not yet been exposed to a wide enough variety of infections. In mild cases of spherocytosis, a splenectomy should not be carried out unless there are significant complications of spherocytosis such as gallstones or leg ulcers.

The spleen can be removed laproscopically (keyhole surgery) meaning faster recovery and a smaller scar compared to traditional open surgery.

Around 10% of people have an accessory spleen, a small piece of spleen-like tissue that is separate from the main spleen. The surgeon should also remove this.

It is possible to have a partial splenectomy, leaving around a quarter of the spleen behind. This helps to maintain the infection fighting function of the spleen. The reduction in symptoms is not as high as a complete splenectomy, so it should only be performed for those with moderate to mild spherocytosis.

Gallstones are a common complication of spherocytosis so, typically, an ultrasound of the gallbladder is performed before the splenectomy to see if gallstones have already formed there. If so, the recommendation is that the gallbladder is removed at the same time as the spleen.

Overwhelming post-splenectomy infection

The spleen has a vital role in the immune system and there are serious risks associated with losing it. There are certain infections that the body cannot fight without the spleen and, untreated, they are rapidly fatal, often within hours. A sudden, severe infection like this is called fulminant sepsis. When it occurs after splenectomy, it can also be called overwhelming post-splenectomy infection (OPSI).

The incidence of fulminant sepsis in those with no spleen is thousands of times higher than for those with a spleen. Even with treatment, an infection like this has a mortality rate of 50%. The highest risk is in the few years following a splenectomy, but the risk is lifelong. If you have your spleen removed, you have approximately a 5% chance of fulminant sepsis in your life.

Some steps are recommended if you have a splenectomy, and failure to follow them is a significant contribution to the infection and mortality rates. The steps include immunisation, antibiotics and seeking medical attention early.

An immunisation schedule should be followed. Both the pneumococcal vaccination and the meningococcal vaccination should be given 14 days before splenectomy and both should be repeated 5 years after the operation. The seasonal influenza vaccination should be given every year and the Haemophilus influenzae type b (Hib) vaccine should also be given, but no revaccination is usually needed.

After a splenectomy, antibiotics should be taken every day for five years. And after that, antibiotics should be readily available to take in case a serious fever develops.

You should also seek immediate medical attention if you have a sudden high fever. Make the urgency of the situation clear to the medical professionals. You might also wish to have a medical alert bracelet, or similar, pointing out that you have no spleen.

In those with no spleen, the parasitical disease babesiosis is life threatening and can cause overwhelming infection. It is caused by single cell organisms that are passed in a tick bite. The same ticks are also the carriers of Lyme disease. The disease is found most frequently in the Northeastern United States, but also in the UK, Ireland and other parts of Europe. When in woodland or grassy areas during May through to September, prevent tick bites by using long clothing and repellant, such as DEET. Inspect for ticks and carefully remove any found as soon as possible.

Consequences

Hemolytic crisis and aplastic crisis

Often someone with spherocytosis will have little in the way of symptoms. Perhaps they feel a little more tired than others. However, this can change dramatically when a hemolytic or aplastic crisis occurs.

A hemolytic crisis is a substantial increase in the rate of destruction of red blood cells (hemolysis). It can be triggered by a variety of parasitical, bacterial or viral infections. For example, both malaria and mononucleosis (also known as glandular fever or mono) can be triggers.

The reason for the increase in hemolysis depends on the type of infection. In a bacterial infection, for example, the immune response increases and this means the spleen has more macrophages (immune system cells that swallow undesirables). This makes the spleen a more hostile environment for spherocytes (the spherical red blood cells), especially as they spend much longer there than normal red blood cells.

The level of red blood cells falls leading to lethargy, weakness, shortness of breath and the other symptoms of anemia. Levels of bilirubin (a break down product of the red blood cells) increase, leading to jaundice, a yellowing of the whites of the eyes and the skin. In a more extreme hemolytic crisis, there can be vomiting, abdominal pain and a tender, enlarged spleen.

An *aplastic* crisis occurs when something prevents the creation of new red blood cells. Some infections have this effect, in particular, parvovirus B19, otherwise known as erythrovirus B19 or fifth disease.

Parvovirus B19 can cause a rash, fever and inflammed joints. The virus attacks stem cells in the bone marrow that would normally mature into blood cells. As a result red blood cell production stops for between 10 and 14 days. In the general population, this causes a small drop in a relatively high red blood cell level. In those with spherocytosis, the drop is larger, because the red blood cells do not last as long, and the starting level is also lower. The effect is much more powerful and it can lead to dangerously low levels of red blood cells.

When levels of red blood cells fall too low, whether due to hemolytic or aplastic crisis, then blood transfusions are needed to provide a boost to the red blood cell levels. Folic acid should be taken. More of it will be required as the body replenishes its stock of red blood cells. In rare cases, immunoglobulin (antibodies) might be given to kill off the underlying infection that was the original cause of the anemia.

Gallstones

Gallstones are a common complication of spherocytosis. They do not inherently cause any symptoms, but they can cause inflammation or blockage which leads to intense pain in the upper right hand side of the abdomen and sometimes vomiting and jaundice.

Gallstones are solidified accretions of matter that form in the gallbladder. There are two types of gallstone, cholesterol and pigment. In the general population, around 90% of stones are cholesterol stones. However, in those with spherocytosis, the stones are typically pigment stones made of bilirubin.

The gallbladder is positioned on the right hand side of the body just under the liver. It has the size and shape of a small pear. It stores and concentrates bile to be released into the digestive tract to help digestion, especially when fatty food is eaten. There are a number of ducts that link the liver (where the bile is produced), gallbladder and digestive tract.

Bile contains bilirubin. Bilirubin is produced when red blood cells are broken down in the spleen. It is a waste product and the liver excretes it, dissolved in the bile. Because of the high rate of red blood cell break down (hemolysis) with spherocytosis, the bilirubin in the bile is more concentrated, compared to the general population. If the bilirubin becomes supersaturated (a higher concentration than the bile can hold) then it crystallizes out to form stones. The stones grow slowly from a small grain up to the size of a golf ball.

The incidence of gallstones, in those with spherocytosis, increases with age from around 40% at age 20 to around 80% at age 70. Under the age of 10, the risk is much smaller, but gallstones still occur in around 5% of cases. The incidence is also related to the severity of spherocytosis, the higher the rate of hemolysis, the higher the risk.

Gallstones only start causing symptoms once they grow to around 8mm in diameter. Those that move out of the gallbladder cause more serious problems.

Gallstones can cause intense pain, called biliary colic. The pain is usually felt in the upper right hand side of the abdomen, but sometimes it is felt in the right shoulder blade, or in both places.

The pain reaches a peak rapidly, within a few minutes, and can be over after 15 minutes, or last for several hours. The pain does not depend on position, and someone with biliary colic will often keep changing position, trying to find a way to reduce the pain. In some cases, the pain is intense enough to cause nausea or vomiting.

Biliary colic is caused by the gallstones irritating the gallbladder or bile ducts. Eating fatty food can bring on an attack, as this is when the gallbladder is more active. Gallstones might irritate by rubbing on the neck of the gallbladder or by moving through a bile duct towards the digestive tract.

Gallstones can inflame the gallbladder (cholecystitis). This causes biliary colic pain, but also fever and nausea. Gallstones block the exit from the gallbladder, preventing the bile from leaving which causes a build up of pressure and a strain on the walls of the gallbladder leading to irritation and inflammation. The stagnant bile can also become infected. Untreated cholecystitis can lead to serious, potentially life threatening complications such as a perforated gallbladder or widespread abdominal infection.

A gallstone can get stuck in the common bile duct (the duct that leads to the digestive tract) and cause a blockage. This is called choledocholithiasis. It causes biliary colic and jaundice (yellowing of the whites of the eyes and skin). Because of the obstruction, the liver is unable to get rid of bilirubin and high levels of this cause the jaundice.

The bile behind the blockage can become infected (cholangitis). This gives symptoms of biliary colic, jaundice and fever. This can be life threatening and requires immediate medical attention. The infection can spread further up the bile ducts to infect the liver.

Diagnosing these gallstone related conditions typically involves using medical imaging such as ultrasound, CT scans or MRI scans.

The treatment for these conditions normally involves strong painkillers for the biliary colic then surgical removal of the gallbladder (cholecystectomy) is advised, to prevent any recurrance. Antibiotics are given if there is any infection and ERCP is used to clear any stones blocking a bile duct.

ERCP (endoscopic retrograde cholangiopancreatography) involves inserting an endoscope (a flexible tube camera) down the throat, through the stomach and digestive tract and into the common bile duct. Through the endoscope, a balloon can be used to expand the duct, freeing the stone, or the stone can be broken up with a high voltage electric spark.

Removal of the gallbladder is one of the most frequently carried out surgical procedures. Typically it is carried out laproscopically (keyhole surgery) as this means faster recovery and a smaller scar compared to traditional surgery.

With no gallbladder, bile constantly enters the digestive tract, rather than a burst of bile when fatty food is eaten. This makes fatty food harder to digest. Some people have more frequent bowel movements, indigestion or chronic diarrhea. Eating smaller meals and less fatty food can help with these symptoms.

There are alternatives to having the gallbladder surgically removed.

Oral dissolution therapy uses bile acid tablets to dissolve the gallstones and contact dissolution therapy uses an injection of solvent into the gallbladder to dissolve them. However, neither of these dissolution therapies are suitable for pigment stones (the ones that occur with spherocytosis) as they only dissolve cholesterol stones.

Extracorporeal shock wave lithotripsy (ESWL) uses acoustic pulses from outside the body to break up stones. This works best on solitary gallstones, especially those that are under 2cm in diameter, but there is a significant chance of the gallstones reforming, especially in those with spherocytosis.

Leg ulcers

Leg ulcers are a rare complication, occurring in around 2% of people who have hereditary spherocytosis.

Typically the ulcers appear on the lower leg, for example on the shin or ankle. They are usually painful and can be several centimetres across. The ulcers do not respond to standard ulcer treatments such as compression via bandages or stockings.

It is not known why the ulcers occur.

Both folic acid supplements and splenectomy (removal of the spleen) have been reported to heal the ulcers, although this can take months.

Extramedullary hematopoiesis

When oxygen levels in the body are lower than normal (anemia), the kidneys produce erythropoietin (also known as EPO). Red bone marrow, found inside bones, contains red blood cell precursors. These respond to erythropoietin by replicating and maturing into red blood cells. This process is known as hematopoiesis. Normally, this increases the number of red blood cells, correcting the oxygen levels.

With spherocytosis, the increased red blood cell production is not sufficient to prevent anemia so the kidney continues to produce erythropoietin. This can cause lumps of red bone marrow to form outside the bones. These are known as extramedullary masses (extramedullary means not in the interior of the bones). These masses provide additional locations for red blood cell production and reduce the level of anemia.

Extramedullary masses can form in a variety of places in the body, but a common site is on the central part of the spine. This can cause lower limb paralysis (paraparesis) and a build up of blood around the lungs (hemothorax).

Extramedullary masses are a relatively rare complication of spherocytosis. They typically occur in those over 45 and occur more often in those with a mild form of spherocytosis because they are more likely to still have their spleen and so be anemic.

The extramedullary masses are often confused with cancerous growths. They are soft, red and bleed profusely when cut. This means that biopsies can cause heavy bleeding, so imaging techniques such as MRI or CT scans should be used for diagnosis where possible.

If the extramedullary masses have not resolved the anemia, then a splenectomy is recommended to prevent the anemia from causing further mass growth.

The masses can be removed by using small doses of radiotherapy (ionizing radiation), but this is only recommended if they are causing a problem. Removing the masses can make the anemia worse, because the masses contribute to red blood cell production.

Hemochromatosis

Hemochromatosis is a condition where the body has too much iron. This can be inherited, in which case it might be referred to as hereditary, primary, type 1 or classic hemochromatosis. It can also happen for other reasons, such as a metabolism disorder or frequent blood transfusions. This is known as acquired, secondary or type 2 hemochromatosis.

Hereditary hemochromatosis is a recessive trait, to inherit it you must get a copy of the gene from both parents. Either parent might only have one copy of the gene and still pass it on, they would be a carrier of the condition, but not suffer from it. About 1 in every 14 people are a carrier for hemochromatosis and about 1 in 250 suffer from it.

The body has no specific mechanism for reducing iron levels. It is not excreted in the urine, for example. However, some iron is lost through fingernail and hair growth and any blood lost takes some iron with it.

The build up of iron is slow, men might be first diagnosed with iron overload between 30 and 50. Whereas, for women it is typically over 50, due to monthly menstrual blood loss.

High iron levels prompt the body to make more ferritin. Ferritin is shaped like a hollow ball and a few thousand iron atoms can be stored inside it. Ferritin provides an iron store for the body.

If the iron overload persists, however, the ferritin molecules get damaged and clump together to form granules of hemosiderin. Ferritin is present in cells around the body, so these iron granules are deposited in a variety of organs.

Wherever the iron is deposited it causes damage. In the liver, it causes cirrhosis and possibly liver failure. In the heart, it can lead to shortness of breath or fatigue and possibly heart failure. In the pancreas, it can cause diabetes. In joints, it can cause joint pain. In the skin, it can cause bronzing.

A frequent treatment used for spherocytosis is blood transfusion, particularly when a hemolytic or aplastic crisis occurs or the spherocytosis is severe. After many blood transfusions, iron accumulates in the body causing secondary hemochromatosis.

Additionally, anemia prompts the kidneys to produce erythropoietin (a biochemical that prompts red blood cell production).

But, erythropoietin also suppresses levels of hepcidin. Hepcidin normally blocks iron absorption, so as the hepcidin levels are lowered by the anemia associated with spherocytosis, the body may absorb more iron than normal.

There is also an increased risk of hereditary hemochromatosis. Although hemochromatosis is normally recessive, if you have hereditary spherocytosis then hemochromatosis can be a dominant trait. You would only need to inherit the gene from one parent, who might only be a carrier. This increased risk of hereditary hemochromatosis remains, even if the spleen is removed.

A simple test for hemochromatosis looks at the level of ferritin in the blood. Normal levels are between around 30 and 300 ng/ml. Treatment is normally advised if this level is over 1000.

A genetic test can determine if any of the known gene mutations for hemochromatosis are present. However, no treatment is required until the ferritin level reaches 1000.

Treatment normally involves regularly drawing about half a litre of blood (phlebotomy) to remove iron from the body, but this increases the anemia of hereditary spherocytosis.

An iron chelator might be given instead. Chelators bind to metal atoms allowing them to be excreted.

Until recently, iron chelation required intravenous drugs to be administered for eight hours, five times a week. However an oral iron chelator that can be taken once a day was approved for use in the US in 2005 and in the UK in 2006. It is called deferasirox (or Exjade). Deferasirox also increases the levels of hepcidin, which blocks iron absorption.

Chelation therapies can take years to reduce iron to normal levels.

Dark urine

Bilirubin is produced when red blood cells are hemolysed (broken down). Because this happens at a higher rate in spherocytosis, levels of bilirubin are higher. Bilirubin is yellow and high levels cause jaundice (yellowing of the skin and eyes).

Bilirubin is excreted by the liver in bile. Bile is held in the gallbladder then released to the digestive system when a fatty meal is eaten. Bacteria in the digestive system break down the bilirubin to urobilinogen, which is colourless. Urobilinogen is then broken down further, by bacteria, to urobilin which is yellow.

Urobilin is excreted in the urine and high levels make the urine a dark yellow, or even brown.

Impact on other conditions

Pregnancy

It is recommended that every pregnant woman take a daily supplement of 400μg of folic acid. This helps prevent neural tube defects in the baby.

Those who have hereditary spherocytosis are often already taking folic acid, with a typical dose of between 1mg and 5mg a day. This folate is given because the higher rate of red blood cell production requires higher levels of folate. If a folate deficiency develops, red blood cell production drops, which can lead to anemia.

The 400μg of folic acid for pregnancy should be taken in addition to any that is being taken for the hereditary spherocytosis, although if 5mg per day is already being taken then this is probably sufficient.

It is likely that women who still have their spleen will become more anemic while pregnant, with a significant increase in the rate at which red blood cells are broken down. In some cases, the anemia can become serious enough to require blood transfusion, both during pregnancy and for a few months after.

After giving birth, the level of anemia slowly returns to its previous point. Studies investigating the impact of this additional anemia on the risk of miscarriage have not found any increased risk.

A woman with a mild form of hereditary spherocytosis might only be diagnosed with hereditary spherocytosis when she becomes pregnant, as a result of this additional anemia.

If the spleen has been removed (splenectomy) then there is not normally an increase in anemia associated with pregnancy. However, there could be problems related to high levels of platelets (small clotting cells). After splenectomy, platelet levels rise because one role of the spleen is to remove old platelets. These high platelet levels normally last just a few weeks, but can, occasionally, remain for years. High platelet levels can cause internal clotting and when this occurs in the placenta, it can cause miscarriage.

If there are high platelet levels during pregnancy then consider taking aspirin to help prevent clots, especially if there is a history of miscarriage.

During pregnancy, it might be useful to prearrange for the child to be tested for hereditary spherocytosis once they are born. This can help diagnose any problems that can occur immediately after birth, such as jaundice.

Malaria

Malaria is a disease caused by plasmodium parasites. Each parasite is just a single cell. The parasites are transmitted to humans by infected mosquitoes when they pierce the skin. The parasites invade red blood cells and multiply there.

The symptoms of malaria are very similar to those of influenza — high fever, sweats, chills, muscle pain, headache, lethargy and possibly vomiting. The first symptoms might appear within two weeks, but it can take several months. Malaria is a serious condition that can be fatal.

There is some evidence that spherocytosis caused by mutations of the spectrin genes restricts the growth of the parasites inside the red blood cell, and this might confer some resistance to malaria.

Some mutations of the band 3 protein gene are known to give malaria resistance, but it has not yet been shown that this is the case for the particular band 3 gene mutations that cause spherocytosis.

The spleen plays a key role in clearing malaria infections, forming immunity and removing infected cells. Spherocytical red blood cells take between 15 and 150 minutes to transit the spleen, rather than 40 seconds for a normal red blood cell. It is possible that because the red blood cells get trapped there, the spleen has more time to act on them and this could confer some extra malaria resistance.

So, if you have spherocytosis then you might be more resistant to malaria, especially if you have just the right type of spherocytosis, but then again you might be no more resistant than the general population. Not enough has been uncovered about malaria to know. This is not something you should rely on.

Because of the role the spleen plays in handling malaria, if you have no spleen then you should take extra care when there is the possibility of being infected: take malaria medication according to the instructions; use mosquito nets; wear long sleeves; use insect repellant.

Atherosclerosis

Atherosclerosis is the thickening of the wall of an artery due to the build up of fatty deposits. It is triggered by oxidation of low-density lipoproteins (LDL). LDL carries cholesterol around the body. Oxidised LDL causes inflammation in the artery walls. The immune response to this brings macrophages (a type of white blood cell) to ingest the LDL, but the LDL filled macrophages clump together to form fatty plaques or rupture, releasing the LDL and continuing the inflammation.

Plaques grow slowly over a period of years. As a plaque grows, the artery wall thickens and eventually this reduces the ability of the artery to carry blood. When this happens in an artery taking blood to the heart, this can lead to heart attack. In an artery taking blood to the brain, it can lead to a stroke.

Bilirubin is a very powerful antioxidant. Higher levels of bilirubin reduce the risk of atherosclerosis by reducing the free radicals that are responsible for the initial oxidation of LDL.

Bilirubin is produced when red blood cells are broken down. Someone with a hemolytic anemia, such as hereditary spherocytosis, has a higher rate of hemolysis (red blood cell break down). This increases the levels of bilirubin, and gives extra protection against atherosclerosis.

After splenectomy, hemolysis returns to normal levels and, as a result, the bilirubin levels also return to normal and this protection is lost.

There also appears to be a connection between free radicals and degenerative neurological conditions such as Parkinson's and Alzheimer's. It is possible that raised bilirubin levels provide extra protection in this area too.

Diabetes

One test for diabetes measures glycated hemoglobin. Hereditary spherocytosis can cause misleading results in this test.

Every red blood cell contains around 250 million hemoglobin molecules. Glucose reacts with hemoglobin to make it glycated. If the levels of glucose that a red blood cell encounters are higher then more molecules of hemoglobin become glycated. Each red blood cell can be thought of as a little glucose meter, accumulating glucose over its lifetime.

In a blood sample there will be young red blood cells that have relatively little glycated hemoglobin and older red blood cells with more. But the average level of glycated hemoglobin across all the different ages correlates to the average level of glucose over the previous months.

In uncontrolled diabetes, the level of glucose in the body is higher than normal, so more hemoglobin becomes glycated.

With hereditary spherocytosis, and other hemolytic anemias, red blood cells do not survive for the normal 120 days. This means that the population of red blood cells is younger and so will not have so much glycated hemoglobin.

As a result, someone with hereditary spherocytosis appears to have lower levels of glucose with this test and this could lead to a failure to diagnose or control diabetes.

Restrictions

Blood donation

If you have hereditary spherocytosis you will not be able to donate blood.

One problem is that you must have a high enough level of hemoglobin to donate. Both the UK and the US adopt minimum levels of 13.5 g/dl for men and 12.5 g/dl for women. This is to protect those giving blood. If you donate half a litre of blood, your hemoglobin level falls by about 1 g/dl. If you already have low hemoglobin, this could make you anemic.

If you have hereditary spherocytosis, then your hemoglobin will likely be too low. Although, if you have had your spleen removed, this may not be the case.

The definitive problem, however, is that the red blood cells from someone with hereditary spherocytosis are more fragile than normal red blood cells and are more likely to be damaged during storage. This potentially reduces the longevity of the red blood cells once they are transfused.

For this reason, regulations for blood donation say that blood should not be accepted from someone with hereditary spherocytosis and this is also the case even if you have had your spleen removed. A similar restriction applies with most other hemolytic anemias.

However, it is possible for someone with hereditary spherocytosis to have blood drawn and stored for later retransfusion. This might be appropriate for scheduled surgery. It has the benefit that a blood type match is guaranteed and also that there will be no risk of infection or allergic reaction.

Military eligibility

Both the US and the UK military have medical eligibility rules that could prevent someone with spherocytosis from enlisting.

The UK armed forces' rules are relatively simple. If you have hereditary spherocytosis then you are ineligible. If you have had a splenectomy to treat it, then you are ineligible because you've had a splenectomy.

The US military rules are more nuanced. If you have anemia then you are ineligible. They classify anemia as a hemoglobin less than 13.5 for men and less than 12 for women. An enlarged spleen (splenomegaly), which is a common symptom of spherocytosis, also makes you ineligible.

The US military rules used to state that you were ineligible if you had had your spleen removed for any reason other than trauma to the spleen. They amended this rule, on the 13th of September 2011, so that having your spleen removed for treatment of hereditary spherocytosis was also acceptable.

Finally, the US military rules make you ineligible if you have had gallstone pain. However, if you have had your gallbladder removed at least six months ago then that is acceptable.

These rules cover all services within the military including army, navy, marines, air force and, in the US, the coast guard.

Exercise

If you have spherocytosis, the problem with exercise is that you can get out of breath or tired more quickly, because you have lower levels of hemoglobin. But, does exercise make things worse?

When exercising, blood is pumped round the body faster. The spleen is a blockage point for those with spherocytosis, so it might be expected that the density of red blood cells in the spleen would go up, which could lead to higher rates of hemolysis and worsen the anemia.

One study looked at the rate of hemolysis during a twenty minute bicycle ride. No extra hemolysis occurred.

Another study reported on endurance atheletes who were going through a period of more intensive training, but yet their performance was declining and they were developing anemia. They were found to have spherocytosis.

These studies seem to be contradictory, but, more likely, moderate exercise has no effect on hemolysis but more intensive exercise is detrimental.

Treatment

Vitamins

There are a couple of vitamins that are potentially important when treating spherocytosis, vitamin B9 and vitamin B12. The body needs both to successfully produce new red blood cells. Because the red blood cells are destroyed at a higher rate in those with spherocytosis, the body compensates by increasing the production of red blood cells. As a result, someone with spherocytosis needs higher levels of these vitamins than someone without.

The methylation and folate cycles

Before we can fully understand the details of how B9 and B12 are used by the body we need to learn about two important biochemical cycles, the methylation cycle and the folate cycle.

The methylation cycle (also called the SAM or SAMe cycle) provides a methyl group to more than forty reactions in the body. A methyl group is a simple combination of one carbon atom and three hydrogen atoms.

The cycle runs through four chemcials. Methionine is transformed to S-adenosyl methionine (SAM). SAM gives up a methyl group to become S-adenosyl homocysteine (SAH) thus driving all those reactions that need a methyl group. SAH is converted to homocysteine which is re-methylated back to methionine. The re-methylation step links to the folate cycle.

The folate cycle is not just a simple loop. There are several loops and various branches. The key chemicals here are all related to tetrahydrofolate (THF).

THF is converted to either 10f-THF or 5,10-methylene-THF. 10f-THF can be converted back to THF, but drives a number of other reactions on the way including the creation of purines (including the letters A and G of the DNA code). The 5,10-methylene-THF is converted to either DHF or to 5-methyl-THF. Both of these are converted back to THF completing the cycle. The conversion of 5,10-methylene-THF to DHF drives the creation of pyrimidines (including the letters C and T of the DNA code). And, as the 5-methyl-THF is converted to THF, it loses its methyl group and converts homocysteine to methionine, carrying out the re-methylation step in the methylation cycle.

Vitamin B9

Vitamin B9 (sometimes referred to as vitamin M) has a number of forms, each with differing chemical structures. The body can use any of these forms to meet its requirement.

Naturally occurring forms of B9 are known as folate. They are not stable, but degrade over a period of days or weeks. There is a synthetic form of B9 called folic acid. It can remain stable over years and is more fully absorbed by the body than natural folate.

Once the body has absorbed the B9, it is converted to DHF (dihydrofolic acid) by the liver and so enters the folate cycle. This conversion process happens at a relatively slow rate in humans.

The liver stores about half of the body's folate. It can release bile containing folate into the digestive system where it is then absorbed and distributed round the body. But, a small amount is lost in the urine in the process, about 1% a day. Folate is also broken down by ferritin (an iron storing molecule). Higher ferritin levels increase the rate of folate break down.

Because of these folate losses, the body needs a supply of B9 to maintain the folate levels.

The folate cycle plays a crucial role in building new cells, such as red blood cells. New cells are normally made by duplicating the DNA in an existing cell to form a new cell nucleus. The cell then splits in two, with one nucleus in each half. As mentioned, one of the functions of the folate cycle is to produce the letters of the DNA code. Without sufficient stock of those letters, DNA replication cannot proceed. The cell grows, as if it will divide, but the division does not happen because a second nucleus does not form.

So insufficient levels of B9 in the diet leads to megaloblastic anemia. There are fewer red blood cells because the cells have not been splitting and they are larger than normal due to the continued cell growth. These oversize red blood cells are called megaloblasts.

Low levels of B9 also increase the risk of cancer because the error rate in DNA replication is higher when there is a shortage of DNA letters.

In pregnant women, B9 deficiency can cause neural tube defects in the unborn baby. This is where the brain or spinal column do not form correctly.

Those with spherocytosis need more B9 because their rate of red blood cell production is higher. As a result, folic acid (the synthetic form of B9) is often prescribed by doctors. A typical regimen would be something in the range of 1mg to 5mg a day. 5mg of folic acid a day is more than ten times the recommended daily intake of folate for a normal adult which is 400μg (0.4mg). Folate is water soluble so excess amounts are excreted in the urine.

If you are taking B9 supplements you may also wish to take B12 supplements because B9 can mask the symptoms of a B12 deficiency (see the Vitamin B12 section below).

Many grain foods are fortified with folic acid: breakfast cereals, bread and other food containing flour. A wide variety of foods have naturally high levels of folate. These include liver, green vegetables (such as broccoli, spinach, lettuce and asparagus), lentils, beans, peanuts, oranges, strawberries.

Folate deficiency can develop relatively rapidly as the body only has enough folate to last a few months before it is completely depleted. Symptoms of deficiency, such as anemia, would appear well before this.

Vitamin B12

Like B9, B12 has a number of different chemical forms. All molecules of B12, regardless of their exact structure contain a single atom of cobalt in the middle. The cobalt gives B12 its other name, cobalamin, and the common forms of B12 are variations on this: cyanocobalamin, hydroxocobalamin, adenosylcobalamin (also called cobamamide) and methylcobalamin.

B12 mediates the link between the folate cycle and the methylation cycle. 5-methyl-THF loses its methyl group, returning to THF. In the process, the methyl group links to the cobalamin to form methylcobalamin. The methylcobalamin then loses its methyl to the homocysteine as part of the methylation cycle.

Without the B12, the folate in the folate cycle builds up in the 5-methyl-THF form. Less folate is then available for the other reactions in the cycle (such as DNA letter synthesis). This is called the folate trap. Similarly, the methylation cycle gets stuck at homocysteine and cannot re-methylate to methionine.

Disruption of the folate cycle leads to the symptoms of folate deficiency, such as megaloblastic anemia (with associated fatigue, pale skin and shortness of breath).

Disruption of the methylation cycle is also serious as it is involved in so many biochemical reactions. In particular, the formation of myelin is suppressed. Myelin is an insulating sheath covering nerve cells and increases the speed at which the electrical signals in the nervous system are sent. So a B12 deficiency can also lead to damage to the nervous system giving numbness, pins and needles, loss of balance, loss of reflexes and personality changes. These symptoms can be irreversible.

High concentrations of homocysteine have also been linked to coronary heart disease and stroke, although the mechanism by which this operates is not yet known.

If you are taking B9 supplements whilst B12 deficient then, despite folate not properly flowing round the folate cycle, folate levels are maintained and there are no symptoms of anemia. The

B9 supplements mask the B12 deficiency. The B12 deficiency might only be noticed once nervous system damage has occurred. So if you are taking a long term B9 supplement (such as folic acid) then you should consider also taking a B12 supplement.

The recommended daily intake of B12 is 2.4µg in a normal adult. This is normally easily achieved in a non-vegetarian diet.

However, the body needs a protein called intrinsic factor in order to absorb B12 in the gut. If the intrinsic factor has been destroyed, by an autoimmune disease for example, then B12 deficiency can easily develop.

Even when there is no intrinsic factor, the body can still absorb a small amount of B12, around 1% of that ingested. So, by taking relatively large supplements of B12 (1mg to 2mg a day), the body's requirement can be met.

B12 is water soluble so excess amounts are excreted in the urine.

Foods that are naturally rich in B12 include liver, fish, seafood and red meat. Plants are not a good source of B12 and so those on a vegetarian diet should also consider B12 supplementation.

B12 deficiency develops relatively slowly as the body typically has stores that can last several years before it is fully depleted.

Antioxidants

Recent research has looked at the effects of free radicals on spherocytes and the effectiveness of antioxidants in preventing hemolysis.

Researchers tested the action of oxidants (free radicals) on red blood cells by adding the oxidants to samples of blood. Spherocytes were damaged more than normal red blood cells. The oxidants affected the cell membrane: damaging fats, altering proteins and creating clumps composed of protein, membrane and hemoglobin.

Some other researchers tested a variety of antiox
blood samples from those with spherocytosis and foun

level of damage due to oxidants was reduced. The antioxidants they used included vitamin C, vitamin E and fermented papaya.

Yet another study treated a group of people who had spherocytosis with fermented papaya for three months and found that their hemolysis reduced and their hemoglobin levels increased by more than 1 g/dl, reducing their anemia.

Gene therapy

There is currently no approved gene therapy for hereditary spherocytosis, but this section discusses how gene therapy might be applied and what research has been carried out in that area.

Gene therapy alters DNA in order to treat disease, for example by replacing a mutated gene with a normal one. It is still experimental, with treatments only now being attempted in animals, or in humans for very serious conditions such as HIV.

One technique uses a retrovirus. These are viruses that normally contain RNA that codes for their construction. They use enzymes to insert a DNA copy of this RNA into the host's DNA. By changing the RNA payload carried by such a retrovirus, custom DNA can be inserted into a host's DNA sequence.

There are several problems that research needs to fully resolve before retroviral gene therapy can become widespread. The DNA must be delivered to the correct place across many cells.

Large pieces of genetic code are harder to deliver as they cannot easily fit inside a retrovirus. Larger viruses are known, but they do not insert DNA into the host DNA sequence, they just release it in the cell.

This would not be suitable for treating hereditary spherocytosis as red blood cells are made from frequently dividing cells in the bone marrow. The DNA needs to be replicated with the cell's existing DNA to be maintained over the long term.

Incorrectly placing the new DNA can cause problems in other genes. One human trial of gene therapy was stopped after patients developed leukemia. The gene therapy needs some mechanism to locate a specific site in the existing DNA to insert the new

DNA. Zinc finger nucleases are a possible mechanism, they use protein structures containing zinc atoms to attach to a specific DNA sequence.

In hereditary spherocytosis, the gene defects are related to red blood cell production. These genes are expressed (used to create proteins that actually do something) very frequently because red blood cells are created very frequently, millions a second. This means that, to be effective, a suitable gene therapy would have to alter the DNA in many cells.

One last thing to consider, is that whilst gene therapy may resolve the problem for the patient, that person may remain a carrier for the disease. In hereditary spherocytosis, the cells that produce red blood cells are not the cells responsible for reproduction.

There is much research to be completed before this becomes a suitable treatment, however there is some research that has been completed on using gene therapy to treat hereditary spherocytosis.

In a test tube, researchers used a retrovirus to alter the DNA of mouse bone marrow cells. The DNA contained a defective gene for ankyrin, a protein that forms part of the red blood cell membrane, and they corrected that defect in at least some of the cells.

This is a long way from a treatment approved for human use, but it gives the first glimpse of the possiblity of a cure for hereditary spherocytosis.

Testing

Full blood count

The full blood count is composed of a number of different tests, each looking at a different aspect of the blood. Together the results give an overview of blood health.

Hemoglobin (Hb or Hbg)

This test measures the level of hemoglobin (the oxygen carrying molecule) in the blood. The normal range is between 13 and 17 g/dl for men and 12 and 16 g/dl for women.

Those with spherocytosis typically have values below the normal range because there are not as many red blood cells. The lower the value, the more pronounced the anemia.

The hemoglobin result is an excellent measure of the level of anemia.

Red blood cell count (RBC)

This test measures the number of red blood cells in the blood. The normal range is between 4.2 and 6.9 trillion per litre for men and 3.5 to 5.5 trillion per litre for women.

Those with spherocytosis typically have values below normal because the body breaks down red blood cells more quickly. The lower the value, the more pronounced the anemia.

White blood cell count (WBC)

This test measures the number of white blood cells in the blood. The normal range is between 3.5 and 11 billion per litre for adults. White blood cells form part of the body's immune system. WBC might fall during an aplastic crisis because the production of blood cells, including white ones, stops.

Platelet count

This test measures the number of platelets in the blood. The normal range is 140 to 450 billion per litre. Platelets help form clots. A low value can prevent blood from clotting, a high value can cause internal clotting.

In those with spherocytosis, platelet counts might temporarily fall during an aplastic crisis or temporarily rise after splenectomy.

Hematocrit (Hct)

This test measures the percentage of the blood's volume that is red blood cells. The normal range is 40 to 60 for men and 35 to 50 for women.

Those with spherocytosis typically have values below the normal range because they have fewer red blood cells.

Mean corpuscular volume (MCV)

This test measures the average volume of a red blood cell in the sample. The normal range is 80 to 100 femtolitres.

Those with spherocytosis tend to be within the normal range or, in extreme cases, below.

Mean corpuscular hemoglobin (MCH)

This test measures the average amount of hemoglobin per red blood cell. The normal range is 25 to 35 picograms per cell.

Those with spherocytosis tend to be within the normal range.

Mean corpuscular hemoglobin concentration (MCHC)

This test measures the concentration of hemoglobin in a red blood cell. The normal range is 31 to 35 g/dl.

Those with spherocytosis typically have values above the normal range. Red blood cells with a high hemoglobin concentration are described as hyperchromic.

Red cell distribution width (RDW)

This test measures the variation in red blood cell width. The standard deviation in the size of the red blood cells is expressed as a percentage of the average size of the red blood cells. The normal range is 11.5% to 14%.

Those with spherocytosis typically have values above the normal range.

Summary

Someone with hereditary spherocytosis would typically have low values for hemoglobin, red blood count and hematocrit; and high values for mean corpuscular hemoglobin concentration and red cell distribution width. A full blood count showing these characteristics would be a strong diagnostic for spherocytosis.

Peripheral blood smear

For this test, a small drop of the blood is smeared across a microscope slide to form a film thin enough to allow individual cells to be seen. The film is stained with a dye and then examined through a microscope.

Normal red blood cells have a paler centre because they are biconcave (disc shaped with a dip in the middle of both sides).

Spherocytes appear smaller, a more intense red and with no paleness in the centre.

If there are a lot of spherocytes in the sample, then this indicates hereditary spherocytosis. The test is not definitive, as spherocytes are seen to some degree in other hemolytic anemias and in autoimmune spherocytosis. But it is simple to perform and useful when taken in the context of other factors, such as family history or other test results.

Osmotic fragility test

The osmotic fragility test measures the ability of red blood cells to retain their integrity in hypotonic solutions. A solution is hypotonic if its salt concentration is lower than that found in the blood, about 0.9% by weight (9 grams per litre).

The test uses around 15 different hypotonic solutions varying in salinity from 0.1% to 0.9%. Each solution has a small amount of blood added to it. In a hypotonic solution, a red blood cell takes in water, lowering the salinity in the cell until it matches the salinity of the solution. This happens through the process of osmosis.

Osmosis is the movement of solvent across a membrane from a lower concentration to a higher concentration. In this case, the solvent is water, the membrane is the membrane of the red blood cell and the concentration of salt in the solution is lower than the concentration in the cell. The water can move across the membrane, but the salt cannot. The water moves to bring the solution and the cell into equilibrium.

When water enters the red blood cell, the volume of the cell increases until the cell bursts. In weaker salt solutions, more water will enter the red blood cells and so more cells will burst. The percentage that burst is measured by shining a particular frequency of green light (540nm) through the solution. Hemoglobin absorbs this frequency. The more red blood cells that have burst, releasing their hemoglobin, the more the light will be absorbed.

The results are typically presented as a graph showing the profile of bursting at different salt concentrations. The equivalent results from a control blood sample are also plotted for comparison.

If the result is given as a single number, then the salt concentration that causes 50% of the red blood cells to burst is often used. This is known as the median corpuscular fragility (MCF). Alternatively, the percentage of burst red blood cells at a particular concentration is sometimes given.

Spherocytes are less able to withstand hypotonic solutions and will burst, even in salinities that are relatively close to blood. This is partly because the red blood cell membranes are weaker, but also because the cells are already spherical and so cannot increase their volume by changing shape, unlike the normal biconcave red blood cells.

Most testing laboratories will incubate the blood in the salt solutions for 24 hours before measuring the amount of bursting. This improves the accuracy of the test. Not all laboratories do this.

There is no widely accepted set of normal results because different laboratories use different testing procedures and this can substantially affect the results. As an example, performing the test at different temperatures can have an effect. This is one reason why a control sample is tested at the same time.

Having said this, after 24 hours, normal red blood cells might burst at around 0.5% salinity whereas spherocytes might burst at around 0.7%.

The test is also used for thalassemia, an inherited anemia that affects the structure of hemoglobin. For that condition, the red blood cells burst at salinity levels even lower than normal red blood cells, the opposite behaviour to the spherocytes.

The osmotic fragility test can only report the presence of spherocytes, it gives no information about why they are there. They could be caused by hereditary spherocytosis, but they could also be caused by other conditions including autoimmune spherocytosis, severe burns or poisoning.

Acidified glycerol lysis test

The acidified glycerol lysis test (AGLT) measures the ability of red blood cells to retain their integrity in an acidic solution of glycerol.

The test uses a slightly acidic solution (pH 6.85) with a low concentration of salt and a high concentration of glycerol. The salinity of the solution is around 0.3% by volume. This compares with a blood salinity of around 0.9%. The glycerol concentration used is thousands of times higher than that found in blood.

A small amount of blood is added. A full blood sample need not be taken, just a drop of blood from a finger or heel prick is sufficient.

Normally, when red blood cells are added to a low salinity solution, water moves from the low salt concentration outside the cell to the high salt concentration inside through osmosis, bringing the concentrations into equilibrium. The cells swell up and eventually burst. In a solution with a salinity as low as 0.3%, red blood cells burst very quickly.

However, it is not as straightforward as that in this test. There is a higher concentration of glycerol outside the cell than inside, so there is a competing osmotic pressure for water to move out of the cell to bring the glycerol concentrations into equilibrium. As a result, the glycerol in the solution slows the diffusion of water into the cell.

Also, glycerol can cross the cell membrane, so the glycerol concentration inside the cell rises over time. As the difference in glycerol concentration decreases, the salt concentration gradient becomes dominant and water diffuses into the cell faster.

Both glycerol and water can enter the cell via two routes. They can diffuse directly through the cell membrane, but they can also enter the cell via special pores called aquaporins.

The red blood cell membrane contains aquaporin-1, which allows both water and glycerol to cross the membrane relatively easily.

Molecules pass through these pores in single file, so when the glycerol molecules pass through these pores they reduce the ability for the water molecules to pass, lowering the rate of water transfer across the membrane.

These various effects combine so that the flow of water into the cell is slowed, but the rate of flow rises over time.

The rate of water influx is measured by shining red laser light (625nm) through the solution. The amount of light that is absorbed is measured.

Small red blood cells scatter more light than large ones. So, as the red blood cells swell, more light gets through, there is less absorption. When they burst, there is no longer a cell to scatter the light, so there is little absorption.

The result of the test is given as the time taken for the light absorption to fall to 50%. This time is usually over 30 minutes for normal red blood cells and less than 5 minutes for red blood cells from someone with hereditary spherocytosis.

The equipment for this test is readily available, it requires only a small amount of blood and it is considered to be highly specific. However, the test requires precise execution to give reliable results.

Some other conditions can give a low result including autoimmune spherocytosis, pregnancy and myelodysplastic syndrome (a disorder of the bone marrow stem cells).

The pink test

The pink test is a slight modification of the acidified glycerol lysis test (AGLT).

The solution that the red blood cells are added to contains not just salt and glycerol, but also sodium azide (NaN_3). The solution is also more acidic than that used in AGLT, with a pH of 6.66 rather than 6.85, and the concentrations of salt and glycerol are also slightly different.

Sodium azide is highly toxic. It has similar properties to cyanide and so must be handled carefully in the laboratory. In this test, it is used at a concentration of 0.01% by weight. Sodium azide acts as a preservative of red blood cells.

The advantage of the pink test over AGLT is that the accuracy of the test does not depend so critically on the acidity of the test solution.

The autohemolysis test

When a blood sample is kept at body temperature (37°C) for 48 hours, some of the red blood cells burst. A higher percentage burst in blood taken from someone with hereditary spherocytosis, compared to normal blood.

Before the blood is incubated at body temperature, it is defibrinated. This means the fibrin is removed. Fibrin is a fibrous protein that helps blood to clot. It is removed to prevent clotting during the incubation. A glass rod (or some other form of glass) is stirred through the blood and the fibrin sticks to it.

After the blood has been incubated, the percentage of red bloods cells that have burst is measured by shining a particular frequency of green light (540nm) through the solution and seeing how much is absorbed. Hemoglobin absorbs this frequency, so the more red blood cells that have burst, releasing their hemoglobin, the more the light will be absorbed.

When normal blood is tested, only about 2%, or less, of the red blood cells burst. In hereditary spherocytosis, the figure is typically 12% to 15%.

Adding sugar (glucose) to the blood before incubation reduces these figures. Under these conditions, for normal blood, there is less than 1% bursting, for hereditary spherocytosis, there is around 3% to 5%. This partial protection of the red blood cells when glucose is present allows hereditary spherocytosis to be distinguished from some other hemolytic anemias, such as pyruvate kinase deficiency where the higher bursting levels remain, even with added glucose.

The cryohemolysis test

In the cryohemolysis test, red blood cells are cooled then the percentage of burst red blood cells is measured. Red blood cells with the membrane defects that occur in hereditary spherocytosis have a higher rate of bursting.

The red blood cells are first placed in a hypertonic solution. A hypertonic solution is one that has a higher concentration than is found in the body. Typically sugar water (sucrose solution) is used in this test. The concentration of sucrose in the body is about 9% by weight. For the test, a concentration of 24% might be used (240 grams of sugar per litre).

The red blood cells are kept in the sugar solution at body temperature (37°C) for ten minutes, then rapidly cooled in an ice bath for ten minutes.

The percentage of red blood cells that have burst is measured by shining a particular frequency of green light (540nm) through the solution and seeing how much is absorbed. Hemoglobin absorbs this frequency, so the more red blood cells that have burst, releasing their hemoglobin, the more the light will be absorbed.

The normal range for this test is between 3% and 15% of red blood cells bursting. Someone with hereditary spherocytosis typically has between 20% and 70% burst.

This test is highly specific for hereditary spherocytosis. Spherocytes caused by other conditions behave like normal cells under this test.

Osmotic gradient ektacytometry

In this test, the deformability of red blood cells is measured as the salinity of the solution that they are in is altered. The resulting deformability profile can be used to diagnose hereditary spherocytosis.

An ektacytometer measures the deformability of red blood cells. There are a variety of designs for ektacytometer, but one might consist of two clear cylinders of different diameters, placed one inside the other, leaving a small space between them.

Red blood cells are extracted from the blood using a centrifuge then added to a clear, viscous (thick) liquid. This liquid is then pumped into the space between the cylinders of the ektacytometer.

One cylinder is fixed and the other rotates about its axis. This causes the viscous liquid to shear: there is a gradient in the speed of the liquid from the stationary cylinder to the moving one. The red blood cells in the liquid are stretched by this shearing.

A laser is shone through the liquid (which is why the cylinders are clear). The light is diffracted by small particles suspended in solution, in this case red blood cells. The smaller the particles, the more pronounced the diffraction.

The laser light forms a circular pattern when both cylinders are stationary, but as the red blood cells are stretched they become larger in the direction of the shearing force, causing less diffraction in that direction. As a result, the diffraction pattern becomes elliptical. The eccentricity (flattening) of the ellipse is measured and this gives a deformability index (DI).

In *osmotic gradient* ektacytometry, the deformability index is measured across a range of salinities. The result is plotted to give a graph somewhat like that shown. The solid line shows a normal profile, the dashed line shows a profile of someone with hereditary spherocytosis.

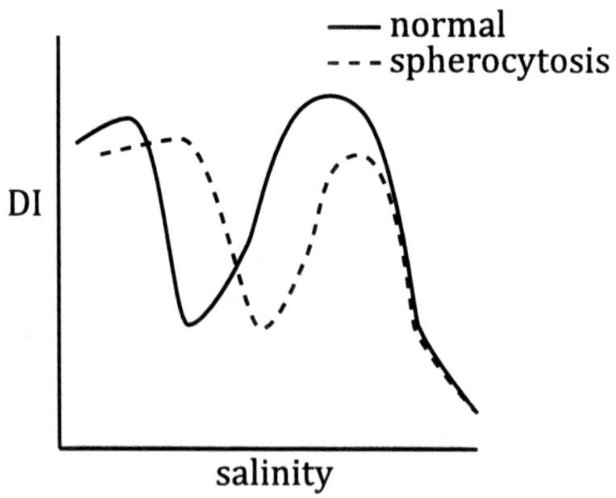

Ektacytometry profile

The deformability hump is lower, narrower and shifted to the right. The more pronounced the change in the profile, the more severe the hereditary spherocytosis.

Information other than the deformability of the red blood cells can be read from the profile. A reduction in maximum deformability implies a reduction in red blood cell surface area. An increase in the salinity at which the deformability reaches half of its maximum implies reduction in red blood cell hydration.

The red blood cells in hereditary spherocytosis are less deformable, have a smaller surface area and are dehydrated.

The profiles for other blood conditions have their own characteristics, so this test can be used to differentiate between them.

The EMA binding test

In the EMA binding test, blood is combined with a fluorescent dye called EMA then passed through a machine that measures the intensity of fluorescence. Hereditary spherocytosis fluoresces with a lower intensity than normal blood. The test is suitable for even very small blood samples.

The full name of EMA (the dye used in the test) is eosin-5-maleimide. It attaches to a group of proteins that form part of the red blood cell membrane. Hereditary spherocytosis has a number of different causes, but they all affect this group of proteins.

The blood sample is mixed with the EMA then kept at body temperature (37°C) for one hour to allow time for the dye to bind to the red blood cell membrane.

The excess dye is removed by briefly centrifuging the sample (spinning it to separate solid from liquid) and rinsing.

The blood cells are then suspended in solution and passed through a flow cytometer.

A flow cytometer pushes a narrow stream of fluid past a laser. Each cell that passes alters the amount of light received by detectors placed around the flowing fluid.

Most relevant to the EMA binding test, the laser light causes the EMA to fluoresce: the laser light is absorbed then re-emited at a lower frequency.

Blood from those with hereditary spherocytosis shows a decrease in fluorescence to around 65% of the intensity that is measured for normal blood.

There are other conditions that give reduced fluorescence, such as CDA-II (congenital dyserythropoietic anemia type II), SAO (Southeast Asian ovalocytosis) and HPP (hereditary pyropoikilocytosis). But, this test can distinguish some of these conditions from hereditary spherocytosis because the intensity of fluorescence is different or there is a characteristic profile of fluorescence (within the population of cells some have one intensity of fluorescence, some have another).

This test is regarded as a highly accurate diagnostic for hereditary spherocytosis.

SDS-PAGE

SDS-PAGE is used to determine the particular protein abnormality in someone with hereditary spherocytosis. Proteins from the red blood cell are added to a gel. An electric field in the gel makes the proteins move. The lighter proteins move more quickly. A stain is used to show the proteins and the result is a sequence of bands showing how far different proteins have moved.

The red blood cells are extracted from the blood using a centrifuge. The blood is mixed with anticoagulant and a salt solution at the same salinity as blood (isotonic solution).

That mixture is spun for just a few minutes in the centrifuge. The red blood cells are dense because they contain lots of iron, which is a relatively heavy element. Because of their high density, the red blood cells settle to the bottom of the centrifuge tube, whilst other parts of the blood stay in the salt solution.

The red blood cells are then burst by adding them to pure water. The water enters the cells through osmosis because there is a high concentration of salt and other solutes inside.

The bursting of the red blood cells releases the hemoglobin into the water, leaving just the cell membranes, known as red cell ghosts.

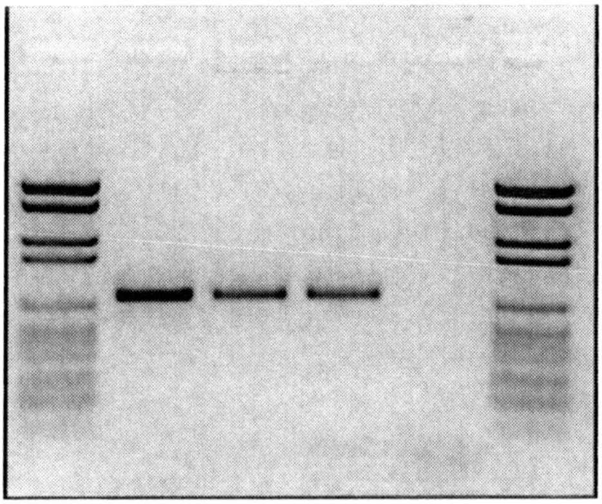

Protein bands in SDS-PAGE

The solution is spun in a centrifuge and the cell membranes settle to the bottom. Hemoglobin dissolves in the water and so stays in the solution.

SDS-PAGE is short for sodium dodecyl sulphate polyacrylamide gel electrophoresis.

The SDS part (sodium dodecyl sulphate) is a detergent. It breaks the three dimensional structure of a protein then attaches along the protein's length. SDS is mixed with the cell membranes. SDS has a negative charge and this gives the SDS coated proteins a negative charge. Longer proteins will have larger negative charges than smaller proteins.

The negatively charged cell membrane proteins are placed at one end of a tray that is filled with polyacrylamide gel. Then an electric field is applied across the gel. The negatively charged proteins are attracted to the positive electrode at the other end of the tray.

Unimpeded, the proteins would all move at roughly the same speed because they all have a very similar mass to charge ratio. However, the proteins cannot move easily through the gel, especially the larger, heavier ones. As a result, the smaller proteins move further than the larger ones, separating proteins out by size.

Finally, a stain is applied to bring out the position of the proteins. Often, Coomassie Blue is used as the stain.

Typically, a mixture of standard proteins of known molecular masses are put into the gel alongside the proteins being tested. This gives a benchmark that can be used to estimate the mass of any other proteins and so identify them.

The relative amount of protein in a particular band can be estimated by scanning light across the protein bands and measuring how much is absorbed at each point. This technique is known as densitometry. The light readings for each band can be compared to give relative amounts of proteins.

A variety of protein deficiencies in the red blood cell occur in hereditary spherocytosis, each caused by an underlying gene mutation. By comparing the ratios of protein amounts against the ratios in normal blood, it is possible to determine which proteins are deficient.

SDS-PAGE can differentiate between the various hemolytic anemias and it is also useful in determining the specific protein abnormality in someone with hereditary spherocytosis. But it is less sensitive for mild forms of hereditary spherocytosis because the ratios of protein amounts are not that different to the ratios in normal blood.

Genetic testing

Hereditary spherocytosis is caused by a mutation in any one of five different genes. The table below shows the code for each gene, the protein that gene normally produces and the location of that gene in the genome (the first number tells you the chromosome).

Gene	Protein	Location
ANK1	Ankyrin	8p11
SPTA1	α-spectrin	1q21
SPTB	β-spectrin	14q23
SLC4A1	Band 3	17q21
EPB42	Band 4.2	15q15

For any one of these genes, there are a number of different mutations that can cause spherocytosis.

Genetic tests are rarely carried out because knowing the precise genetic mutation that has caused the spherocytosis has no implications for treatment. It may be useful, however, to determine whether the spherocytosis is dominant or recessive, when that is not clear from a family history.

Testing newborn babies

There are two reasons to test a newborn baby for hereditary spherocytosis: one of the parents has hereditary spherocytosis or the newborn has significant levels of jaundice.

If one of the parents has a dominant form of hereditary spherocytosis then each child has a 50% chance of inheriting the gene. In this situation, newborn babies should be tested for hereditary spherocytosis.

Jaundice is a yellow colouring of the skin and eyes caused by raised levels of bilirubin. It is quite common in the first few days of a newborn baby's life, with around half of newborns having some level of jaundice. The liver processes bilirubin to be excreted in the bile, but a newborn baby's liver takes a while to reach full effectiveness.

About 5% of newborns have jaundice severe enough to require treatment. This is usually due to an elevated level of hemolysis, most commonly because of an incompatibility between the mother's blood group and the baby's.

This incompatibility can be confirmed by a positive Coombs test. For this test, antibodies are added to a blood sample and, if the blood cells clump together, then the test is positive.

Other blood conditions, such as hereditary spherocytosis, are normally only considered once there is a negative Coombs test. Around 1% of newborns with a high level of jaundice have hereditary spherocytosis.

Levels of bilirubin above 30 mg/dl are dangerous in newborns and can cause brain damage (kernicterus) because the blood-brain barrier is not fully developed, so the bilirubin can cross to the brain.

Levels can be reduced by using light therapy. Bilirubin breaks down in light and just placing the baby under an intense blue light can break down bilirubin in the body.

The blood composition of newborn babies is different to that of an adult. This makes testing for hereditary spherocytosis in newborns more difficult.

A newborn has more, bigger red blood cells and this means hemoglobin levels are higher. The appearance of the peripheral blood smear is unusual and the osmotic fragility ranges are different. However, more sophisticated tests such AGLT or the EMA binding test are still effective.

Serious jaundice occurs in approximately 90% of newborns who are diagnosed with hereditary spherocytosis in the first week of life.

The following table shows how often newborns with hereditary spherocytosis require blood transfusion due to anemia in the first few months of life.

Transfusions	Frequency
No transfusion necessary	30%
One transfusion	40%
More than one in the first months of life	20%
Severe HS requiring ongoing transfusion	10%

Test accuracy

Tests are not always accurate. Sometimes a test will report someone has hereditary spherocytosis when they do not, or fail to report they have it when they do.

The percentage who have hereditary spherocytosis, that the test correctly identifies as having it, is known as the sensitivity. The percentage who do not have hereditary spherocytosis, that the test correctly identifies as not having it, is known as the specificity.

A higher sensitivity means the test misses fewer cases. A higher specificity means that fewer people are diagnosed as having hereditary spherocytosis when they do not have it.

A perfect test would have 100% sensitivity and 100% specificity.

The first step towards a diagnosis for hereditary spherocytosis is usually a full blood count, a peripheral blood smear and a Coombs test.

A full blood count showing lower hemoglobin, raised MCHC (mean corpuscular hemoglobin concentration) and raised red cell distribution width would be a strong indicator of spherocytosis.

This would be further confirmed by spherocytes in the peripheral blood smear and a negative Coombs test would discount autoimmune spherocytosis.

There are a number of different tests that can then be used to confirm a diagnosis of hereditary spherocytosis. They vary in sensitivity, specificity, simplicity, availability and cost. Simplicity, availability and cost are related: simple tests are generally cheaper and more available.

The most accurate tests, with sensitivities above 95% and specificities to match, are AGLT, cryohemolysis, EMA binding and osmotic gradient ektacytometry. Often the equipment for EMA binding and osmotic gradient ektacytometry is not available (a flow cytometer and ektacytometer respectively). AGLT requires precise execution to generate reliable results.

Slightly less accurate, with sensitivities between 80% and 90% are the pink test, incubated osmotic fragility test and autohemolysis test. The pink test and the autohemolysis test are relatively easy to carry out and the pink test has the additional advantage of needing only a small amount of blood making it suitable for newborn babies. The osmotic fragility test is a relatively old test that has been superseded.

Overall, the cryohemolysis test is a good choice for a confirmatory test as it can be carried out easily, without sophisticated equipment and is a highly accurate test.

Glossary

Accessory spleen: a small piece of spleen-like tissue that is separate from the main spleen.

Allele: a gene variant.

Anemia: lowered levels of oxygen in the blood.

Ankyrin: a structural protein of the red blood cell membrane.

Antibody: a large protein that attaches to antigens and neutralises them.

Antigen: a foreign molecule or cell.

Aplastic crisis: temporary halt to red blood cell production.

Atherosclerosis: thickening of an artery wall due to the build up of fatty deposits.

Autoimmune: relating to the immune response of the body against itself.

Autosomal: an inheritance pattern not linked to gender.

Biconcave: the shape of normal red blood cells: a disc with a dip on both sides.

Biliary colic: pain caused by gallstones.

Bilirubin: a biochemical that results from the break down of red blood cells.

Centrifuge: laboratory equipment that spins samples forcing solids to settle out of suspension.

Chromosome: a large molecule of DNA containing many genes. There are 23 chromosomes in normal humans.

Cobalamin: vitamin B12. The folate cycle is hampered without it.

Coombs test: a test that adds antibodies to blood to detect autoimmune hemolytic anemias.

Cytoskeleton: the supporting structure of the cell.

Dominant: an inheritance pattern where an allele overrides another.

Ferritin: a molecule that the body uses to store iron.

Fibrin: a fibrous protein that helps blood to clot.

Flow cytometer: laboratory equipment to automatically count and analyse components of a blood sample.

Fluorescence: the emission of light by a substance after it has absorbed light at a higher frequency.

Folate: vitamin B9, used to build new red blood cells.

Folate trap: a situation where folate cannot move round the folate cycle due to a vitamin B12 deficiency.

Folic acid: a synthetic form of folate.

Free radical: a molecule with an unpaired electron and thus highly reactive.

Fulminant sepsis: a sudden, severe infection.

Gallbladder: an organ that stores and concentrates bile to be released into the digestive tract, helping digestion.

Gallstone: a solidified accretion of matter that forms in the gallbladder.

Hemochromatosis: a condition where the body has too much iron.

Hemoglobin: the oxygen carrying molecule.

Hemolysis: the break down of red blood cells.

Hemolytic crisis: a significant increase in the rate of hemolysis.

Hetrozygous: relating to two different alleles.

Homozygous: relating to two matching alleles.

Hypertonic: of a higher salinity than found in the blood.

Hypotonic: of a lower salinity than found in the blood.

Hypoxia: a condition where the oxygen levels in the blood are so low that demand cannot be met.

Intrinsic factor: a protein responsible for the absorption of vitamin B12.

Jaundice: a yellowing of the skin and whites of the eyes due to high levels of bilirubin.

Kernicterus: brain damage caused by high levels of bilirubin. This only occurs in newborns.

Lymphocyte: a type of white blood cell responsible for generating antibodies.

Macrophage: a type of white blood cell that swallows antigens and damaged red blood cells.

Megaloblast: an unusually large red blood cell.

Myelin: an insulating sheath covering nerve cells.

Osmosis: the movement of solvent across a membrane from a lower concentration of solute to a higher concentration of solute.

Osmotic fragility: the extent of red blood cell break down in hypotonic solutions.

Phenotype: the observable characteristics of an individual.

Phlebotomy: drawing blood.

Plaque: a fatty deposit on an artery wall.

Platelet: small cells that help blood to clot.

Recessive: an inheritance pattern where one allele cannot override another.

Red pulp: a fine mesh of blood vessels in the spleen that filter the blood.

Reticulocyte: an immature red blood cell.

Solute: a dissolved substance.

Spectrin: a structural protein of the red blood cell membrane.

Spherocytes: spherical red blood cells. Normally blood cells are biconcave.

Spleen: an organ that is part of the immune system and also filters old red blood cells.

Splenectomy: surgical removal of the spleen.

Splenomegaly: an enlarged spleen.

Transfusion: the process of adding blood to the body via an intravenous drip.

White pulp: part of the spleen that is involved in aspects of the immune system.

CPSIA information can be obtained at www.ICGtesting.com
Printed in the USA
LVOW062332190313

325028LV00028B/1055/P

9 780957 194502